H₂O Workouts®

Pool Ball Fun

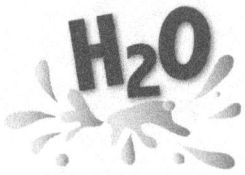

Francine Milford, LMT

H2O Workouts® Pool Ball Fun
Copyright© 2012 Francine Milford

Photographs by Paul, Larry and Francine Milford

ID: 978-1-105-88397-2

Caution
The techniques, ideas, and suggestions presented in this book are not intended as a substitute for proper medical advice. Any application of the techniques, ideas, and suggestions in this book is at the reader's sole discretion and risk.

Please consult your health care provider before beginning this or any other exercise program.

Fitness for the Next Generation

As more people are recognizing the need to live healthier and better lives, they have begun to set goals on how they will achieve and maintain a healthy body through proper nutrition and balanced work schedules.

Before long, the entire face of a typical aerobic class was changed as millions of people attempted to find a way to add exercise into their daily lives. Classes ranged in levels from easy senior workouts and classes for pregnant women to the high paced, high intensity Boot Camp classes.

Soon, many people were experiencing injuries from pushing their bodies too long and too far. When people are impatient to see results, they tend to exercise for long hours in a short period of time. Overuse injuries are one of the most common injuries found in the fitness industry.

Now most facilities offer Tai Chi, Qigong, Yoga and Pilates for people who want a good workout without the stress and strain of strenuous exercise.

The Great Equalizer

I call the water environment, the Great Equalizer. When I have taught water aerobic classes I would have ladies enter the water on crutches and even one came to class in a wheelchair. Once in the water, you could not tell the ladies apart. In the water environment, everyone is equal and everyone can receive a workout that is right for them and their fitness level.

In this book I will be sure to list exercises in **LEVELS**. If you are a beginner, then please stick to **Level One** exercises. As your body becomes familiar with the moves and becomes stronger, then move on up to **Level Two** and **Level Three**. Remember, don't overdue your workouts or you risk injuring your body and not being able to exercise at all.

Principles of Water Exercise

The water environment offers two important natural occurring effects to the water routine: buoyancy and resistance. Buoyancy is the property of being able to float. Buoyancy is also the power of a liquid to keep objects afloat; in this case, that object is you.

It is the natural ability of water to act as a cushion and in so doing, it protects you joints from injury, strain and re-injury. Many rehabilitation centers use the water environment in their treatment sessions.

While in the water environment, people can perform exercises they otherwise could not on land. Among these exercises are jumps, leaps, jumping jacks and pivots. Amazingly enough, the ability of water to be buoyant also allows water to provide resistance to water aerobics. Through changing direction, adding speed, or using longer levers, the water can provide a complete and thorough workout.

The water environment can become a natural total body workout. The more you put into your workout, the more you will receive from it. The faster you move, the harder the exercise becomes.

Water aerobics is also the perfect environment for those who are overweight or suffer from physical injuries. When you stand in water that is chest deep, you weigh only 10% of your normal body weight.

The water environment is also the great place to practice your golf or tennis swing. Even dancers and weight trainers can use the resistance in the water to build up muscles in a safe way.

Tips for a Safe Workout

Do's and Dont's
- Do wear aqua shoes or aqua socks
- Do keep head in alignment of the spine.
- Do exercise in water that is of correct depth for you.
- Do relax and breathe slowly and deeply.
- Drink plenty of water before, during, and after exercising.
- Consult with your doctor before you begin exercising.
- Work at your own fitness level.
- Stop exercising if you feel faint, dizzy, nausea, or shortness of breath.
- Don't smoke or drink alcohol while exercising.
- Don't make fast, uncontrolled movements of the head or trunk in any direction.
- Don't use extreme range of motion.
- Don't use quick, jerky movement.
- Don't exercise with food or gum in your mouth.
- If you feel tired-stop
- For safety, there should be a lifeguard on duty during your workout or invite a friend to exercise with you.
- Never drink alcohol before, during, or immediately after a water workout.
- Perform your exercises in water that is chest high.
- Wait at least 1-3 hours after eating before working out
- When you enter the water that is cool, be sure to beginning walking, jogging, or bouncing right away to get your circulation moving.
- Always begin exercising slowly and then working up to more strenuous, energetic moves.
- Remember-Have fun!

Workout in Water

Warm-ups

As in any exercise program, it is important to prepare the body for the work that you are planning to put it through. We call this preparation, the Warm-Up.

In the Warm-Up you will increase the flow of blood to each and every muscle of the body. In this way, you will greatly reduce the risk of injury.

Warm-up exercises are usually gentle and slow activities that normally last 5 to 15 minutes. During this phase all the muscles and joints should be put through simple movements beginning with small range of motions and then increasing to larger, or full, range of motion.

In a typical land aerobic or workout class, we begin simply with marching in placing. The same holds true for water aerobics. In this chapter we will include several muscle groups that you will need to be sure you warm-up before beginning a water aerobics class. For some, this may be all the exercise that you can do in one day and if so, that is perfectly okay. What is important is move and stretch your body as often as you can throughout the day to keep it limber and lubricated.

When I received my certification in Aquatic Exercise, we practiced many types of water walking. Following a 3 to 5 minute warm-up exercise (such as marching in place) you could do some of the following walking exercises for the next 20-45 minutes:

- Walk forward and backwards
- Walk to the right and Walk to the left
- Walk in a big clockwise circle, then walk in a big counter-clockwise circle
- Walk on your toes

- Walk on your heels
- Walk like a crab sideways bouncing from flat feet with knees bent and open to the sides of your body.
- Walk forward and backward punching the water.
- Walk three steps and hop for one step.
- Do the Congo step in the water.
- Do the Bunny hop in the water.
- Do the Electric Slide in the water.
- Do your favorite Western Two Step in the water.
- Alternate between fast and slow walking to add intensity.
- Do the Soldier Walk, otherwise known on Goose Stepping
- Do Karate Kicks
- Walk doing knee lifts forward and front leg lift backwards
- Do Pendulum Swings with your legs side to side
- Do the Rocking Horse forward and backwards and change legs.
- Do Hamstring Curls forward and backwards.
- When stretching muscles in the warm-up phase it would be good if you could hold each stretch for at least 10 seconds (30 seconds is optimal).

Stretching

When performing the warm-up exercises and stretches, you should be able to feel slight warmth within your body. This is good and signals that you are preparing your body for the more vigorous workout that is to follow. The muscles that are stretched during the warm-up phase are the muscles that will be worked through the aerobic phase.

The Toe and Ankle Warm-ups

Some warm-up exercises and stretches can be performed inside, or at poolside, before you ever enter the water. If you find it difficult to spend more than 20 minutes in the water, then performing the warm-up stretches before entering the water may be a good idea.

Toes and Ankles

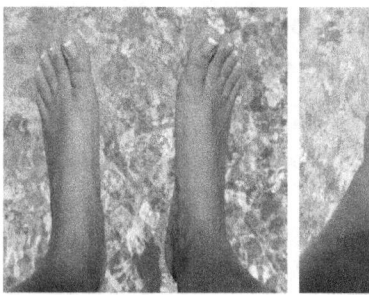 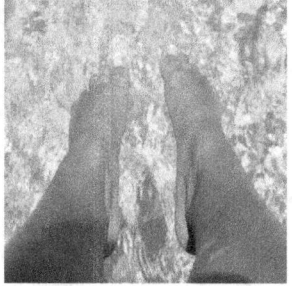

To Do: Slowly point your toes towards you as far as you comfortably can, hold, and release, now press your toes away from you, hold and release. Do this exercise for eight repetitions.

Toes and Ankles

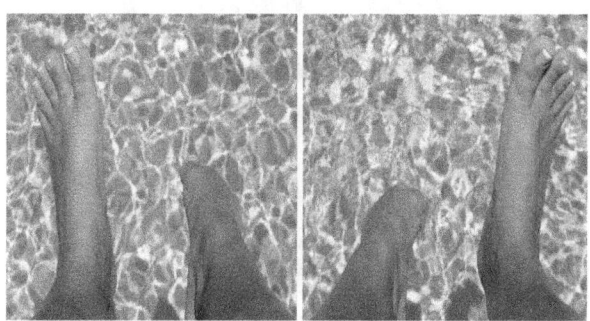

To Do: Alternate between flexing and extending your feet. Press your right toes away from your body while you bring your left toes toward you body, hold for a few seconds, and then relax the stretch. Now, bring your right towed toward your body and press your left toes away from your body at the same time. Continue to alternate between your two feet in this way for a total of eight repetitions.

If you are sitting poolside, you can perform this exercise either outside of the water, or inside of the warm. The choice is up to you.

Toes and Ankles

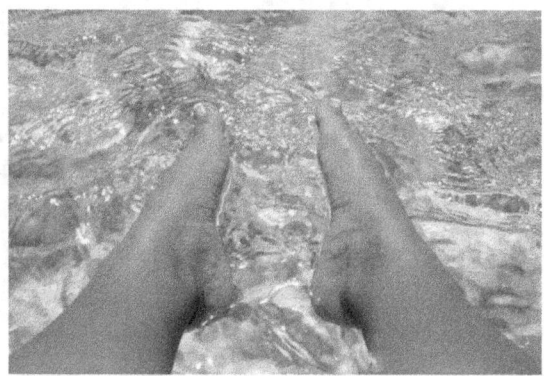

To Do: In the exercise above you will press the soles of your feet towards each other, hold for a few seconds, and then relax the stretch. Perform this stretch for eight repetitions.

Now, press the soles of your feet away from each other. Repeat for a total of eight repetitions. Bring your focus to each of the soles of your feet and do not crunch your toes or fold them over one another.

You will also be feeling a stretch in the front part of your leg, this is the anterior tibialis. When this muscle is not properly warmed up and stretched, many people suffer from Shin splints.The front of your leg should begin to feel warm, as well as, your ankles.

Toes and Ankles

Feet Swinging

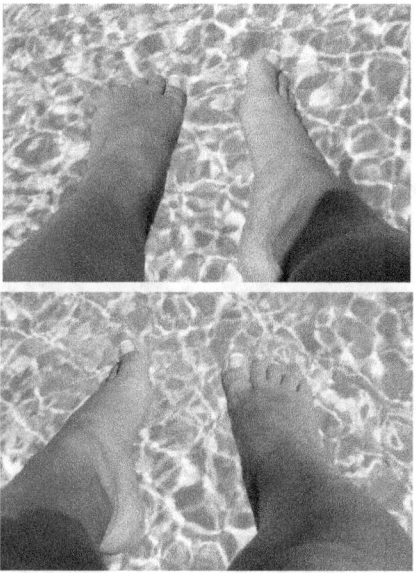

To Do: In the exercise above you will swing your feet to your right, hold for a few seconds, then swing your feet to the left, hold for a few seconds, and then relax. Perform these feet swinging exercises for eight repetitions. Have fun with the exercise feeling the resistance of water on your feet.

Toes and Ankles

Circles

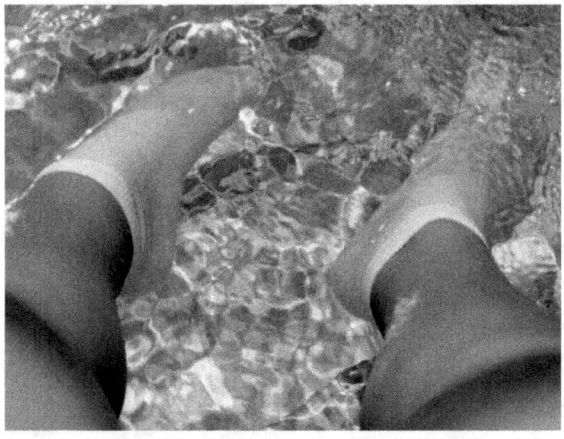

To Do: Using both feet at the same time, begin to move your feet in a circle clockwise. Begin by making eight small circles and then continue to enlarge each circle until you are making eight of the largest circles you can with you feet. Repeat the same exercise this time creating the smallest circles we can

Warm-ups for the Neck

Like the warm-ups for the toes and ankles, warm-ups for the neck can be performed on land before you enter the water environment. Do not push these stretches beyond what your physical capabilities are. Stretches should not be painful. If they are, stop immediately and consult with your primary health care provider.

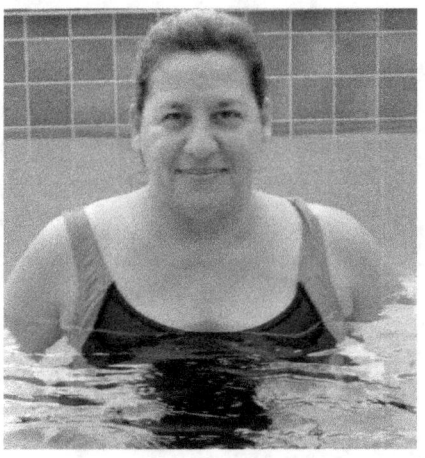

Starting Position

The starting point for the neck exercises will begin with the head in a neutral position as is shown in the diagram above, on the left. Keep you gaze in front of you at a slight angle downward. Be sure to breathe normally.

Neck Warm-ups

Neck

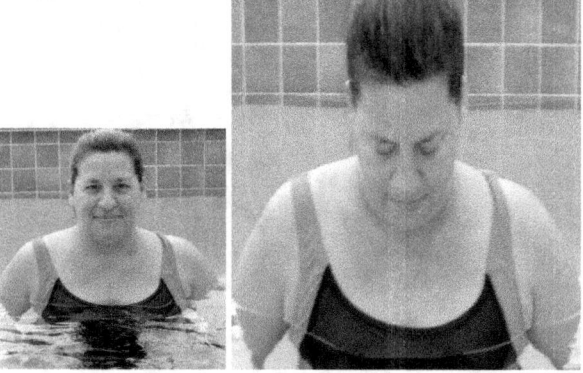

To Do: With your head in the starting position take a nice deep slow breath in. As you exhale, slowly allow your head to fall forward touching your chin to your chest (note: if you cannot touch your chin to your chest, this is alright, don't force the movement.)

Now, slowly inhale and begin to return your head to the starting position. Repeat this exercise for a total of eight repetitions.

Neck

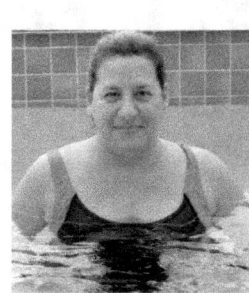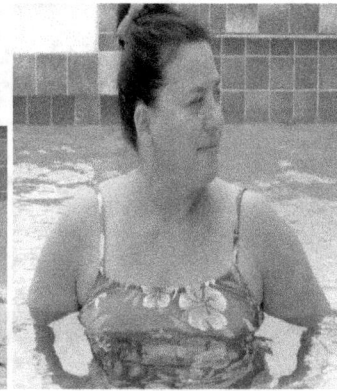

To Do: With your head in the starting position take a nice deep slow breath in. As you exhale, slowly turn your head to left aligning your chin to over your left shoulder (note: if you cannot align your chin to over your shoulder, this is alright, don't force the movement.) Now, slowly inhale and as you exhale, begin to return your head to the starting position.

With your head in the starting position take a nice deep slow breath in. As you exhale, slowly turn your head to right aligning your chin to over your right shoulder (note: if you cannot align your chin to over your shoulder, this is alright, don't force the movement.) Repeat this exercise for a total of eight repetitions.

Neck

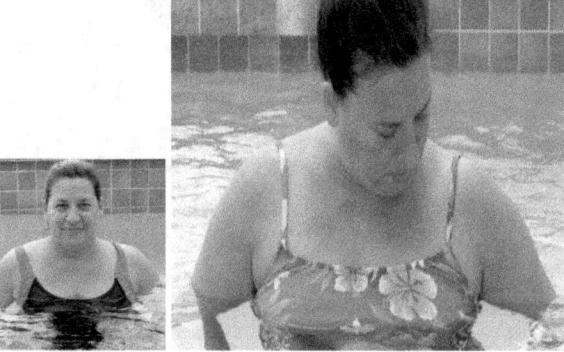

To Do: With your head in the starting position take a nice deep slow breath in. As you exhale, slowly allow your chin to drop to the left to a point that is located half way between the center of your chest and your left shoulder (note: if you cannot touch your chin to your chest, this is alright, don't force the movement.) Now, slowly inhale and as you exhale, begin to return your head to the starting position.

With your head in the starting position take a nice deep slow breath in. As you exhale, slowly allow your chin to drop to the right to a point that is located half way between the center of your chest and your right shoulder (note: if you cannot touch your chin to your chest, this is alright, don't force the movement.)

Repeat this exercise for a total of eight repetitions.

Neck

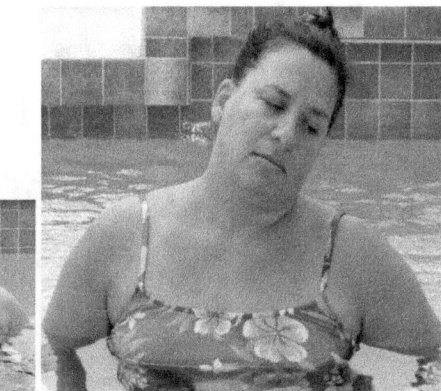

To Do: With your head in the starting position take a nice deep slow breath in. As you exhale, slowly allow your left ear to drop to your left shoulder (note: if you cannot touch your ear to your shoulder, this is alright, don't force the movement.)

Now, slowly inhale and as you exhale, begin to return your head to the starting position.

With your head in the starting position take a nice deep slow breath in. As you exhale, slowly allow your right ear to drop to your right shoulder (note: if you cannot touch your ear to your shoulder, this is alright, don't force the movement.)

Repeat this exercise for a total of eight repetitions.

Neck

Head Rolls

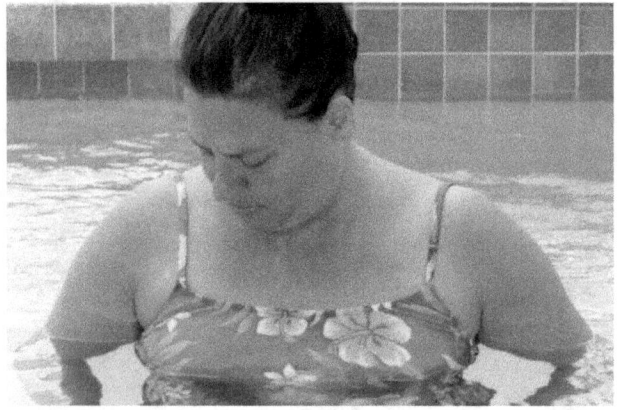

To Do: Imagine that your nose is like the hands of wall clock. The numbers of the wall clock are right in front of your face. Take a nice deep slow breath in and as you slowly exhale you will begin with your nose in the twelve o'clock position. Moving clockwise outline the numbers of the clock from 3, to 6, to 9, and ending back at the top at the number 12 position. Repeat for eight repetitions.

Now, repeat the above exercise, this time moving counter clockwise beginning at the 12 position moving down to the 9, 6, 3, and back to the top 12 position. Repeat for eight repetitions.

Warm-up for the Shoulders

Shoulders

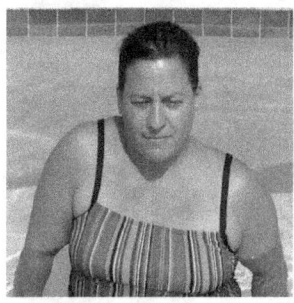 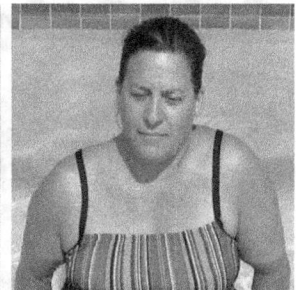

To Do: Bend your knees slightly with arms down at your sides. Standing perfectly straight, inhale and bring your right shoulder up to your right ear and hold. As you exhale release the shoulder back down to starting position. Remember-do NOT bring your ear down to meet the shoulder. Repeat for a total of 8 repetitions. Now, inhale and bring your left shoulder up to your left ear and hold. As you exhale, relax and return to the starting position. Repeat for a total of 8 repetitions.

Alternating Shoulders: Inhale and bring your right shoulder up to your right ear and hold. Exhale and relax the shoulder back to the starting position. Inhale and bring your left shoulder up to your left ear and hold. Exhale and relax the shoulder back to the starting position. Repeat for a total of 16 repetitions.

Shoulders – Shrugs

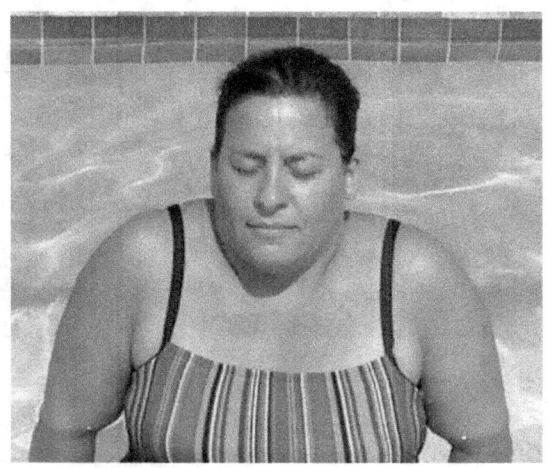

To Do: Inhale and bring both of your shoulders up to your ears and hold for a few seconds. As you exhale, allow both shoulders to relax and return to the starting position. Continue for a total of 16 repetitions. This is a great exercise to do throughout the day to reduce stress.

Shoulders – Circles

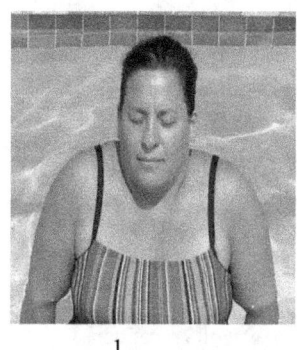

1

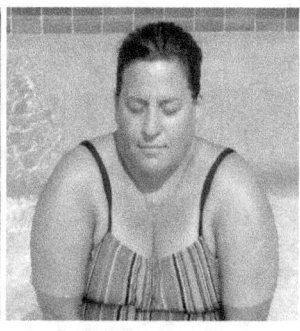

2

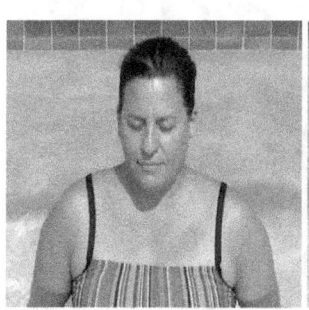

3

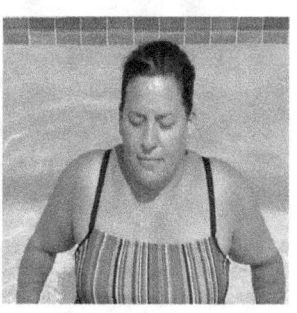

4

To Do: Inhale and bring both shoulders up to your ears (1) and as you exhale allow the shoulders to push forward (2), then down (3), then back behind you (4) forming a circle. As you inhale again pull the shoulders back up to your ears and repeat the circle of exhaling and allowing the shoulders to drop to the front, down to the sides and to the back before returning up to the ears again. Repeat for a total of 8 repetitions.

When finished, repeat this exercise, this time inhaling and bringing the ears up to the shoulders and as you exhale, allowing the shoulders to drop towards the back, down to the sides, up to the front and back up to the ears in the next inhalation. (4-3-2-1). Repeat for a total of 8 repetitions.

Pectorals, some arms and shoulders

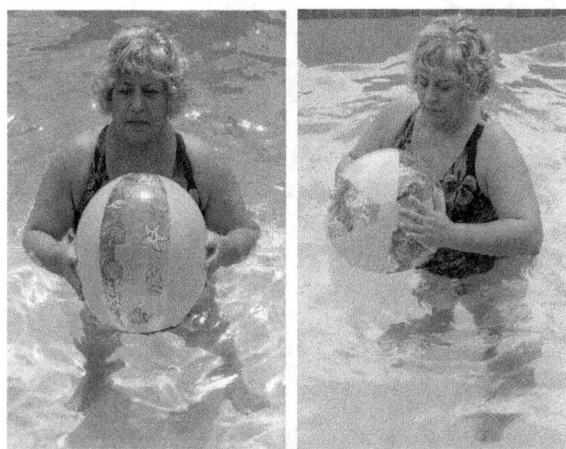

Starting Position

To Do: Place your hands on the sides of the ball. Keep your feet flat on the bottom of the ball with your knees slightly bent. Inhale, and as you exhale bring your hands, and the ball, together in front of you. Squeeze, count to 10 and release. Repeat for a total of eight repetitions.

Arms and Shoulders

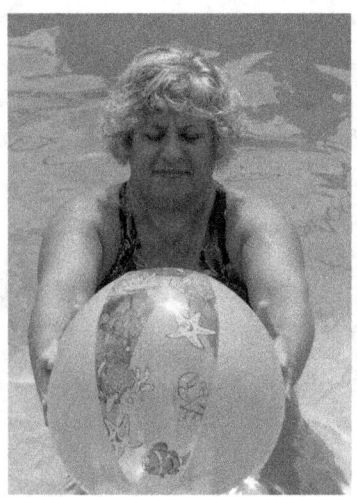

To Do: Begin with feet firmly planted on the bottom of the pool and your knees slightly bent. Place both of your hands on the ball in front of you at shoulder width apart. Inhale, and as you exhale push the ball away from your body as far as you can. Inhale and bring the ball back to your chest. Continue to exhale and push the ball away from you and inhale while bringing the ball to your chest. Repeat for a total of at least eight repetitions.

Arms and Shoulders

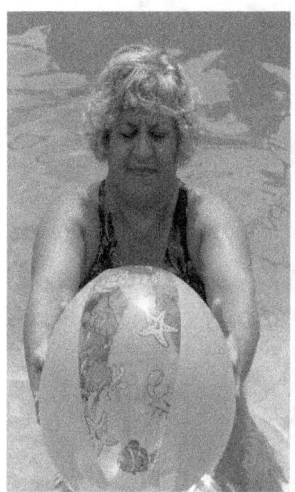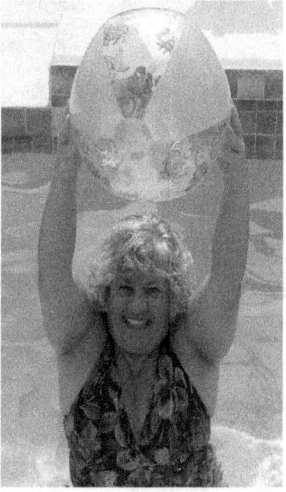

To Do: Begin with feet firmly planted on the bottom of the pool and your knees slightly bent. Place both of your hands on the ball in front of you at shoulder width apart. Inhale, and as you exhale lift the ball over your head as far as you can. Inhale and bring the ball back to your chest. Continue to exhale and push the ball away from you and inhale while bringing the ball to your chest. Repeat for a total of at least eight repetitions.

Arms and Shoulders

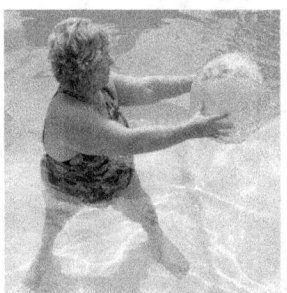

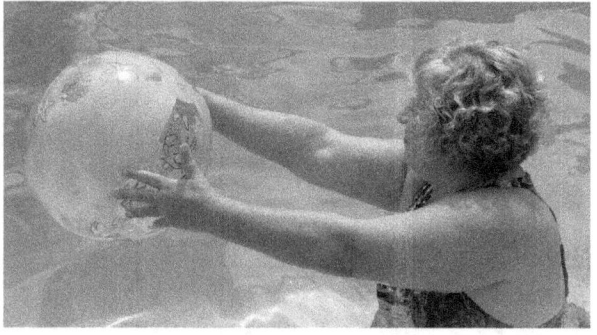

To Do: Hold the ball between your hands above the water. Inhale and as you exhale turn your body to the right, hold for a few seconds, inhale and as you exhale, slowly release back to the starting position. Repeat for a total of at least eight repetitions on the right and then do eight repetitions on the left. Alternate turning right and left for eight repetitions.

Arms and Shoulders

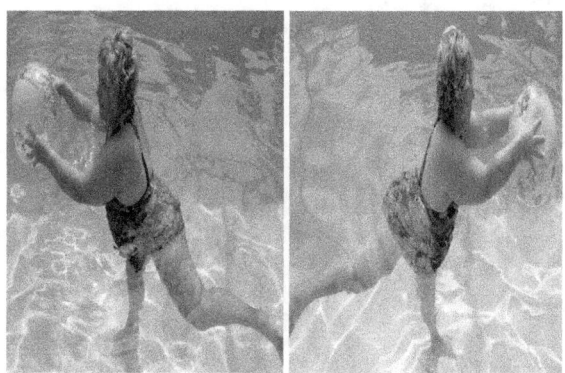

To Do: Keep your feet planted firmly on the bottom of the pool with knees in a relaxed position. Hold the ball between your hands and above the water like in the previous exercise.

Inhale and as you exhale, turn your body to one side. Hold for a few seconds and bring one left up as high as you can. Feel a good body stretch. Inhale again and as you exhale return to the starting position and repeat on the other side. Do not overextend your body to the point of discomfort.

Do a total of eight repetitions.

Warm-up for the Wrists

Note: If you have any wrist problems or injuries-please consult your health care provider before beginning these exercises.

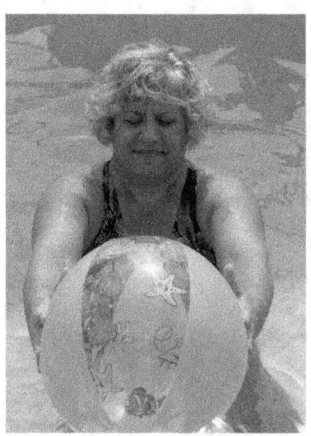

Starting Position

To Do: Stand with both feet on the ground, knees relaxed. Hold the ball between your hands just above the water. This is your starting position.

Wrist Twist

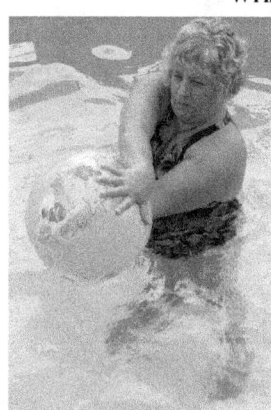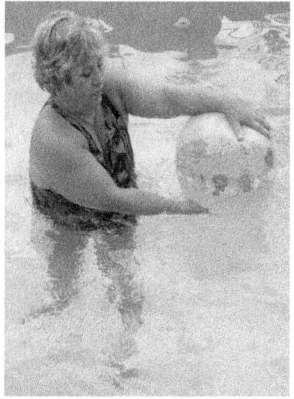

To Do: Begin the following exercises in the starting position as shown in the previous picture. Extend both of your arms straight out in front of your body holding the ball above the water. Keep your arms straight but do not lock your elbows.

Move your hands as shown in the pictures above. Start with one hand over the other and then rotate to the other over the hand. Repeat for a total of eight to sixteen repetitions.

Side Wrist Twist

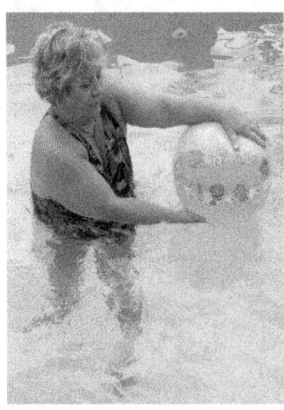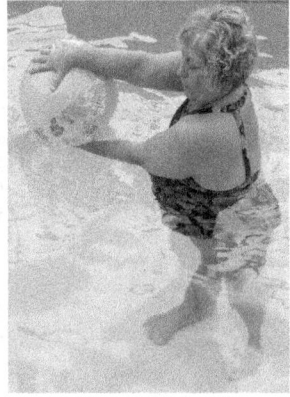

To Do: Extend both of your arms straight out in front of your body. Do not lock your elbows. If this is uncomfortable, just relax your arms and do the best that you can. Take a nice slow, deep breath and at the same time turn your body to the side as shown in the photograph above, while keeping your arms extended away from your body. Inhale and as you exhale return to the starting position. Repeat for a total of eight repetitions.

Basic Water Moves

Knee-ups

Knee-ups – Level One

Begin with both of your feet firmly planted on the bottom of the pool. Now, as you are balancing yourself, lift your right knee up as high as you can. Do not go over a 90 degree angle. Press your right foot back to the bottom of the pool and straighten out your leg. Do this for a total of 8 repetitions and repeat the whole exercise on your left leg. Work at a nice, steady, and slow speed. Take your time. Work up to 25 repetitions on each leg.

Knee-ups - Level Two

Walk slowly forward and backward from one side of the pool to the other side. The faster you walk, the more intense the workout will be. You can call it 'Power Walking' if you like. Try to keep the pace slow and steady so that you can keep your balance without too much stress on your body. Move your arms through the water at your side as you try to walk briskly forward and backward. Don't overdo this exercise as you will quickly discover that it will tire you out and increase your heart rate very rapidly.

Knee-ups - Level Three

1. **Alternate Knee Lifts**-For this exercise you will alternate between lifting the right knee and lifting the left knee. The exercise will be "Right knee up, right knee down, Left knee up, left knee down." Repeat this for a total of 16 repetitions. Alternate the rate of speed that you are using to perform this

2. **Running in Place**-Should you be able to alternate the speed of your leg lifts enough, you will be able to start running in place. Do this for 30 seconds working up to a minute or more. To add variety and intensity, practice running at different rates of speed for a great workout.

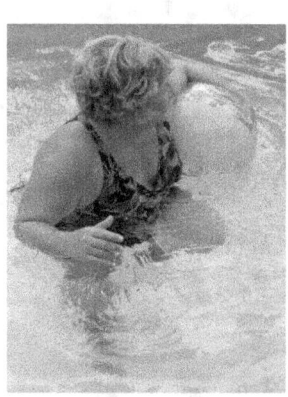 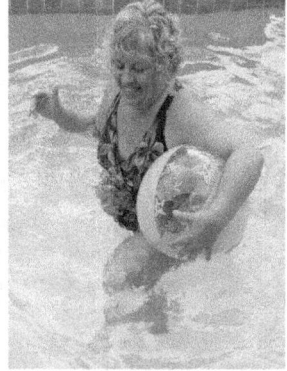

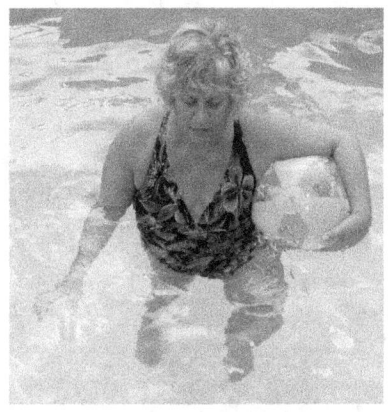

3. **Running with Movement**-Add direction. Run in a circle as fast as you can. Do this for 8 repetitions. Run in a clockwise circle, then switch direction and run in a counterclockwise circle. Do this for several repetitions on each side.

Alternating Knee Lifts

Single Knee Lifts- Level One

Begin with both of your feet firmly planted on the bottom of the pool. Lift your right knee up toward the left side of your body and bring your ball over to touch the right knee. Return the right foot back down to the bottom of the pool and straighten up your body. Repeat for 8 repetitions, and then repeat the entire exercise using the left knee and the right side of your body.

Alternating Knee Lifts - Level Two

Alternate lifting the right and left knees. The exercise will go like this: "Left knee up towards right side of body, right knee up towards left side of body, and straighten up. You will do this for a total of 16 repetitions. Work up to 25 repetitions.

Alternating Knee Lifts - Level Three

You will now do the alternate knee lifts as described in Level Two but at a faster rate of speed. You will feel like you are running and you feet may not come fully down on the bottom of the pool. To add variety and intensity, alternate between slow and fast rates of speed, this will help to build up your heart rate. If you like, you can move forward and backward while doing this exercise.

Front Leg Lifts

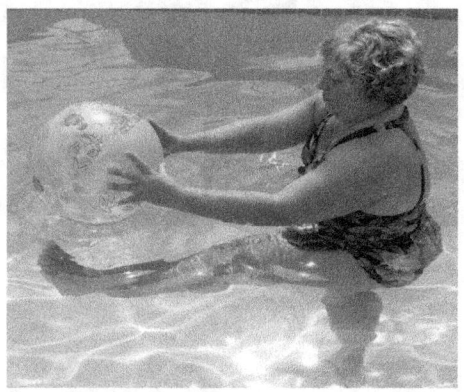

Level One-Begin with both feet planted firmly on the bottom of the pool and with your knees soft. Now, inhale and bring your left leg straight up in front of you as high as you comfortably can, hold for a few seconds, and then as exhale, bring your leg back down to the starting position. You can try to touch your foot to the ball. Do a total of eight repetitions and then repeat exercise on the other leg.

Level Two- Alternate lifting your right and left leg. Continue alternative the front leg lifts for a total of 16 repetitions.

Level Three- Add speed, hopping from right to left leg. Move forward and backward while alternating front leg lifts.

Side Leg Lifts

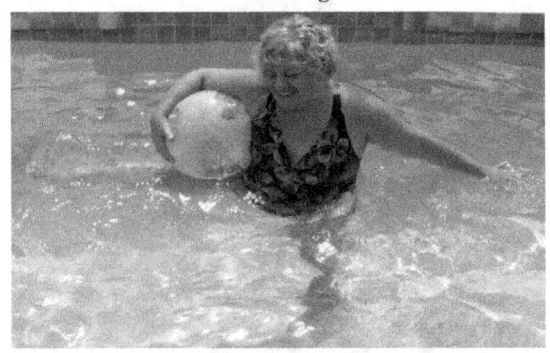

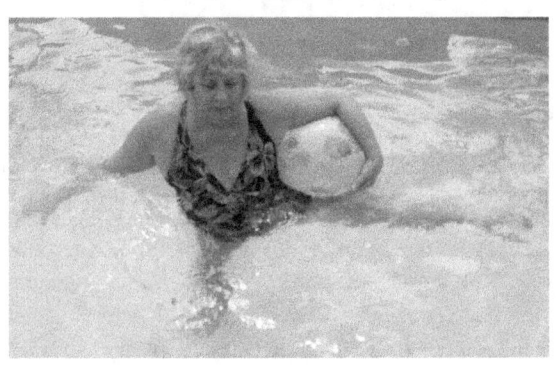

Side Leg Lifts – Level One

Plant both of your feet firmly on the bottom of the pool and keep your knees soft. Now, inhale and lift your right straight up at your side as high as you comfortably can, hold for a few seconds, and then exhale and release the leg back to the starting position. Repeat for a total of eight repetitions. When finished, repeat the entire exercise on your left leg

Side Leg Lifts - Level Two

Plant both of your feet firmly on the bottom of the pool and keep your knees soft. Now, lift your right leg up as far as you can to your right side and return to the starting position. Then, lift your left leg up as far as you can to your left side and return to the starting position. Repeat alternating between the right leg and the left leg for a total of 16 repetitions.

Side Leg Lifts – Level Three

Add speed to the exercise shifting rapidly between the right and left leg lifts. Move forward, backward, and sideways from one end of the pool to the other. You can vary your speed and even add a double hop on one foot.

Play some upbeat music while you are exercising and 'dance' to the music while you are doing your water workout. Match your speed and movements to the songs you have chosen to alleviate any boredom you may suffer from exercise. With music, you see the time fly by very quickly. Be sure to pick music that makes you want to move and if you can sing along with the words, all the better.

Inner/Outer Thigh Work

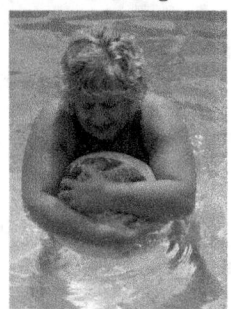

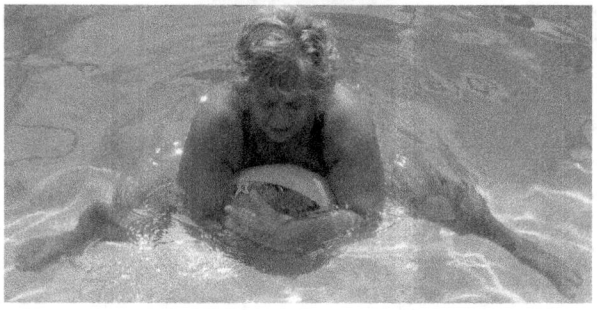

To Do: Begin by leaning forward comfortably on your pool ball. Inhale, and as you exhale press the ball down into the water, spread your legs as far apart as you comfortably can as shown in the above picture on the right, and jump up in the water. Exhale and bring your legs back together again. Do eight times.

Triceps

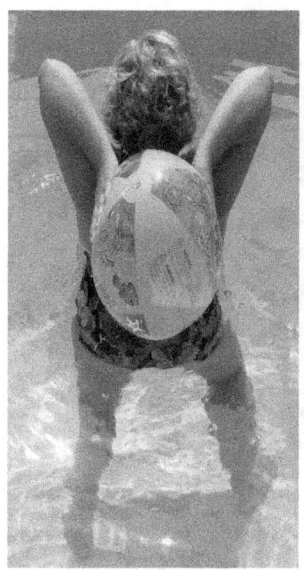 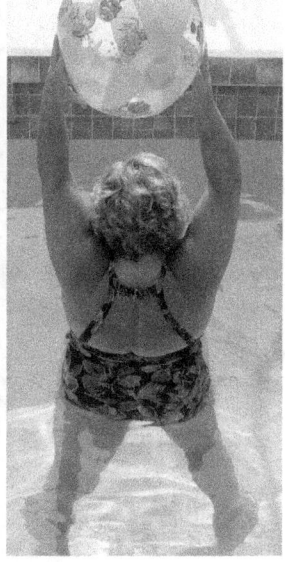

To Do: Stand with your feet apart. Hold the ball between your hands and lift your straight arms up overhead. Now bend your elbows and allow the ball to rest on your back. This is the starting position. Now inhale. As you exhale, lift your arms straight overhead (as if you were going to through ball). Inhale and bend your elbows back to the starting position. Repeat for eight repetitions.

Quadriceps

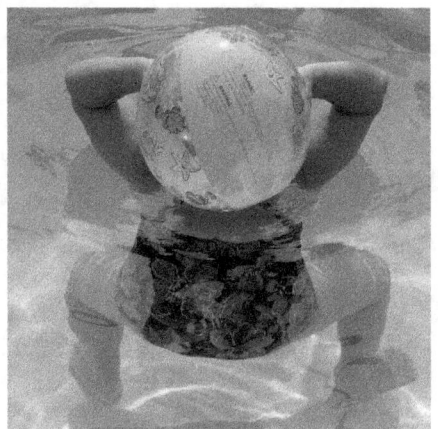

Starting Position

To Do: With feet firmly on the bottom of pool and legs apart, inhale and squat down.

Triceps and Quadriceps

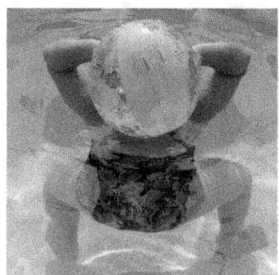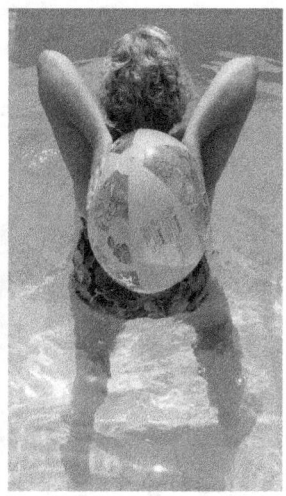

Level One-Inhale and squat down. As you exhale, return to standing position by pushing off the bottom of the pool with your heel. Do at least eight repetitions.

Level Two-You can additional intensity by adding triceps work (extending arms as you stand and flexing while squatting). You can work on speed by squatting slow or fast. You can also squat and lift one knee up when you stand and then when you squat and stand again-you can lift the other knee up.

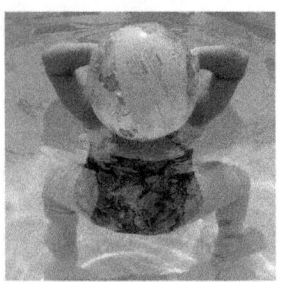

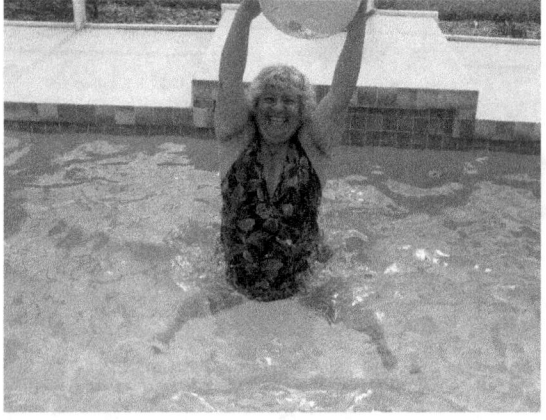

Level Three-Squat like in the previous exercises, but you will add a hop out of the water as if you were shooting a basketball into a hoop. Repeat for a total eight repetitions.

Abdominal

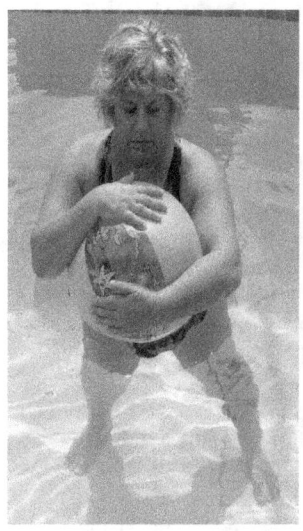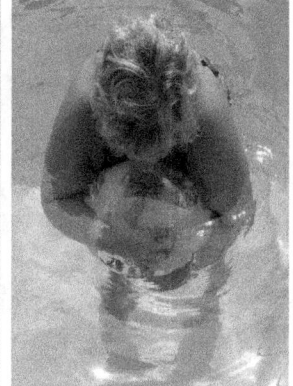

To Do: Begin this exercise as shown in the photograph on the top left of the page by grabbing your ball between your hands and leaning slightly forward.

Inhale and as you exhale, roll your body over the ball allowing your feet to come off the bottom of the pool. Inhale and return to starting position. Repeat for eight repetitions.

Stretches

Shoulder Stretch

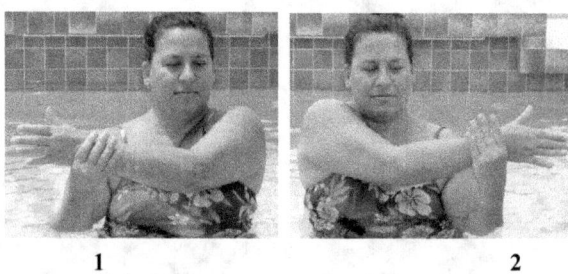

1   2

To Do: Begin the cool down by bringing your straight left arm across the front of your body and gently grasp your left wrist with your right hand (as shown in picture #1). Gently press the left arm toward your right arm.

Be sure to keep your hips and body straight and looking forward. Do not force the stretch and be sure to inhale and exhale freely and easily. Release the arm.

Now, take your straight right arm and bring it across the front of your body and gently grasp your right wrist with your left hand and press the arms towards your left arm (as shown in picture #2). Release the arm. Repeat on both sides for an additional two more times.

Shoulder Hug

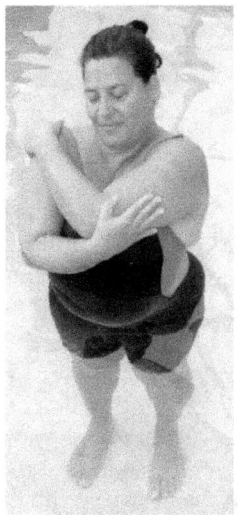 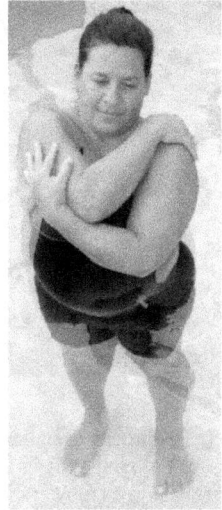

To Do: A great shoulder stretch in the 'hug'. Just wrap your arms around each other and give yourself a big hug. Inhale and exhale freely and easily.

Release your hug and switch your arms around and give yourself another big hug. Inhale and exhale freely and easily. Repeat the hug for an additional two more times on each side.

Stretch

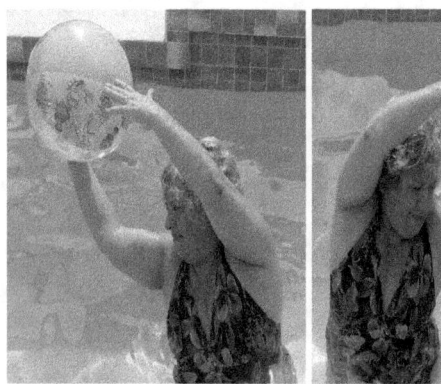

To Do: Begin this exercise by standing with feet flat on the bottom of the pool and shoulder width apart. Inhale and reach your arms straight upward from your body while holding the ball between your hands. Exhale and bring arms to one side of the body.

Inhale and as you exhale return to the starting position. Repeat on the other side. Perform this stretch a total of eight times on each side.

Hip Stretch

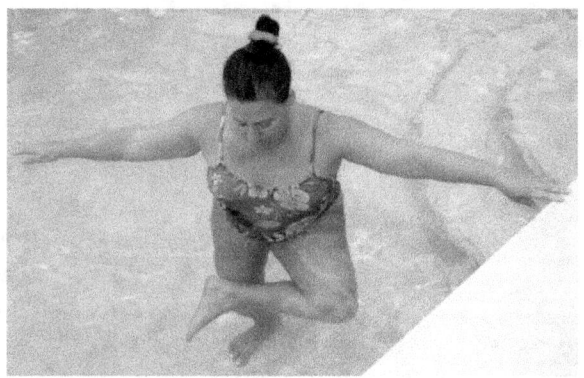

To Do: Stand with both of your feet planted firmly on the bottom of the pool shoulder width apart. Bend your left knee and bring your left up the front of your body and place it just above your knee.

Now, as you exhale, slowly bend your right knee and allow yourself to sink into the water as far as you can comfortably go. Hold, and then release into starting position. Repeat this exercise on the other side using your right foot on your left thigh.

To add more depth to this hip stretch exercise you can do the following: As you sink into the water as far down as you can go, hold that position and lift up off the heel of your foot.

Cool Down

Cool Downs are a series of movements that are used after an exercise class as a means to return the heart rate back to its normal pre-exercise rate. The more you exercise, the stronger your heart and lungs will become and the shorter the period of time it will take for the heart rate to return to normal. If you need help in adapting any of these exercises to your own specific limitations, just drop me an email at RevReikiND@cs.com and we can discuss options.

Cool Down

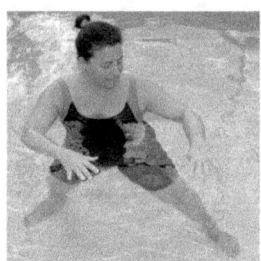 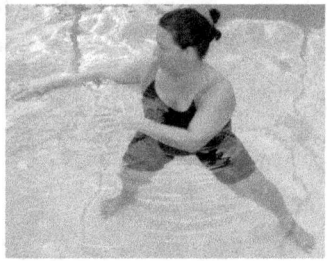

To Do: You can add mindfulness and breath to this cool down exercise. To do this exercise, spread your legs apart as far as you comfortably can to maintain your body's balance in the water.

Place your hands, palm down, at the very top of the water and pretend that there are flower petals floating on the top of the water. Gently push the flower petals to the left and then to right trying not to disturb the petals, or the water.

About the Author

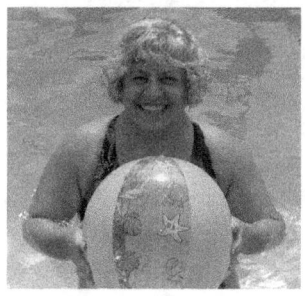

Francine Milford has had a very long career in the Fitness Industry. Working for more than 25 years in a variety of sports and exercise related classes, she is also an avid walker and enjoys reading a book audio tape while bicycling around the neighborhood.

A national and state licensed massage therapist and personal trainer, Francine has achieved certifications through the YMCA S.A.F.E. Aerobic Program, AEA Aquatics Exercise Association, ESA Exercise Safety Association, and AFAA Aerobics Fitness Association. She has also received the Tai Chi for Arthritis Certification having studied under Dr. Paul Lam, as well as, 180 hours of professional training in Tai Kwan Do. She has taught such classes as Kick Boxing, Bench Stepping, Low Impact Aerobics, High Impact Aerobics, Basic Floor and Senior Aerobics and all types of Water Aerobic classes.

As a fitness specialist, Francine has been hired to lead classes and workshops at offices, condo organizations, clubs and private groups. Having spent the last 20 years working with the senior population, Francine has developed exercises that are both safe and effective for those with physical limitations. Visit online at www.H2OWorkouts.com or at www.ReikiCenterofVenice.com.